Raising Ducks & Geese - Homesteading Animals

For Meat, Eggs & Feathers! Includes Duck & Game Recipes For The Slow Cooker

By
Norman J Stone

Guest Blogger on www.planterspost.com

Published By

www.deanburnpublications

2 Titles In 1 Volume Including..

Homesteading Animals (2) – Delightful Ducks

Homesteading Animals (3) - Gourmet Geese

Copyright

Copyright © 2014-24, Norman J Stone

All rights reserved. Copyright protected. Duplicating, reprinting or distributing this material without the express written consent of the author is prohibited.

The information contained in this book is for general advice only. Users should always consider local regulations concerning the keeping, rearing, or consumption of animals.

The statements contained herein have not been evaluated nor approved by the US Food & Drug administration.

While reasonable attempts have been made to assure the accuracy of the information contained within this publication, the author does not assume any responsibility for errors, omissions or contrary interpretation of this information, and any damages incurred by that.

The author does not assume any responsibility or liability whatsoever, for what you choose to do with this information.

The cooking and other techniques described in this publication are for your general guidance only.
Use your own judgment.

Table of Contents

Title 1 – Delightful Ducks 9
    Introduction: 10
    Duck Care 13
    Ducklings 14
    Feeding Time! 16
    Good Shelter 19
    Duck Health 22
Preparing For The Table 27
Popular Domestic Duck Breeds 32
    Indian Runner Duck 32
    American Pekin Duck 33
    Crested Pekin: 34
    Khaki Campbell 35
    Rouen Duck 36
    Muscovy 37
    Buff Orpington 38
    Bantam Duck Breeds 39
    Silver Appleyard Miniature 41
    East Indie Bantam 41
    Traditional Call Duck 42
Title 2 - Gourmet Geese! 43
    Introduction 44
Beginning With Geese 46

- Popular Breeds 50
  - Emden (or Embden) 50
  - Brecon Buff 52
  - White Chinese 53
  - African Goose 54
  - Pilgrim 55
  - Toulouse 56
  - Roman 58
- Caring For Geese 60
  - Shelter: 60
  - Pasture & Feed: 62
  - Gosling Care: 65
- Keeping Healthy Geese 68
  - Fowl Cholera: 68
  - Aspergillosis: 69
  - Nematodes (Roundworms): 69
  - Lameness: 70
  - Coccidiosis: 71
- Preparing For The Table 72
  - Preparation: 72
  - Plucking: 73
  - Evisceration: 75
  - Cooking Goose 76
- Tasty Duck & Game Recipes 78
- **Authors Note:** 86

Title 1 – Delightful Ducks

Homesteading Animals (2): Delightful Ducks

Rearing Ducks For Meat & Eggs

Includes Duck & Game Recipes For The Slow Cooker

By
Norman J Stone

A special thanks to F. A. Paris for the game recipes 'borrowed' from 'Slow Cooking Heaven'
(Copied by Permission)

www.deanburnpublications.com

Introduction:

When you picture in your mind a typical Homesteading, there are many animals that will probably take 'front stage' in your ideal vision; and I have little doubt that Ducks and Geese will be seen happily splashing around a small pond or water feature – if not…why not!

Along with Chickens; Ducks and Geese - perhaps even Turkeys - can play a major role in the drive to become self-sufficient and to lead a more 'Holistic' lifestyle.

In many ways Ducks are even easier to raise than chickens, are great foragers amongst the vegetables as they seek out slugs and other creepy-crawlies (watch out for your prize plants though!) Certain breeds can supply an abundance of highly nutritional (and large) eggs, whilst others can be raised specifically for their meat.

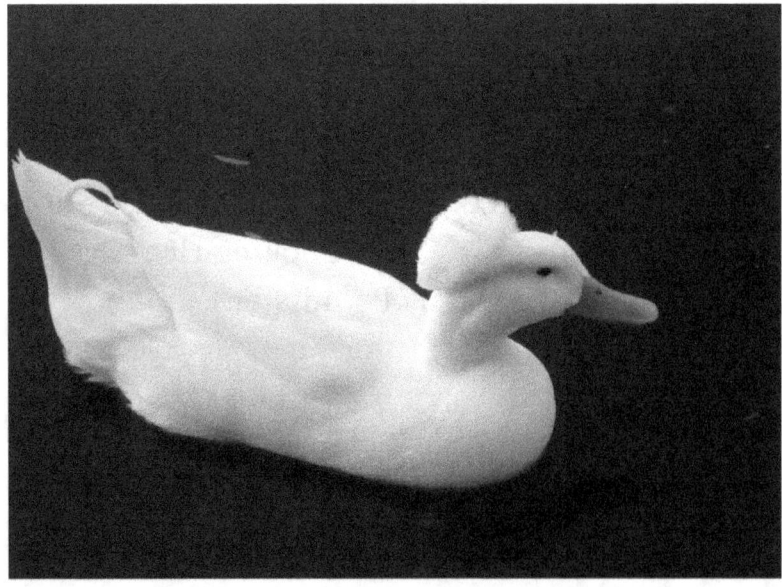

Some of the more ornamental bantam ducks such as the miniature Appleyard or the Black East Indie, are just great to marvel at as they happily waddle around the steading; kids love them, and they are not as messy as their larger counterparts – they also make quite good layers!

Geese on the other hand, are great for their meat and eggs, but also as an early warning system! Nothing can sneak past a couple of Chinese Geese; there is even a prison in north-eastern Brazil that uses them as an early alarm system!

Back in the day, when I was a 'young-un' my first job was to look after the poultry, which included ducks, geese, turkeys, hens and even a few golden pheasants!

Out of them all the ducks were my favourites, and I could watch them for ages as they splashed around in anything that resembled a pond – no matter how shallow.

I had a dozen white Chinese Pekins at the time, and they loved nothing more than feed time, when I would fill up their small pond with clean water and they would all noisily fight to get prime spot.

True, they did create an awful mess in the process, but it was worth it just to watch them having such fun. It was at that time I developed a great liking for duck eggs: Stronger than chickens eggs, and they make a great omelette!

Needless to say I wasn't so keen when it came to eating them, and I learned my first painful lesson about rearing animals for food – NEVER name your animals; unless you are keeping them as pets – more on this later.

I hope you enjoy this introduction to rearing Ducks, and if not already doing so, will consider these marvellous and versatile animals for your own Homestead.

Duck Care

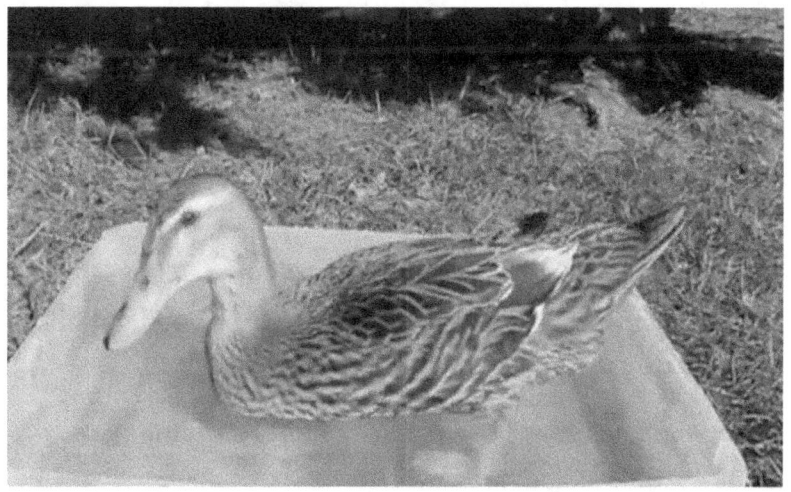

In general, Ducks are very undemanding animals, and as long as a few rules are adhered to, they are generally very healthy and robust; able to withstand a variety of weather conditions and temperatures.

As an addition to the Homestead or farm, they are an invaluable source of meat, highly nutritious eggs and even fluffy down for your pillow. They also make great pets for the kids, and will follow you around and be as devoted in their own way as the family dog – in many cases outliving their canine friends, as they can live up to 20 years or more!

With all that said, here are a few basic steps to put into place if you want to get the best out of your Ducks and keep them healthy and happy.

Ducklings

If you are rearing your own ducklings via a broody duck (or hen) then there are certain precautions that must be taken.

Firstly, it takes 28 days for the eggs to hatch after the parent has started to brood (35 days for Muscovy ducks).

The broody duck on the nest must be kept in a quiet, safe environment, where she will not be disturbed and possibly abandon the eggs prematurely.

When the ducklings have hatched, be sure to stop them immersing themselves in water for at least one month; this allows time for the preening gland to operate. Bathing before this time will simply mean that the chick will catch a chill or drown, as it is not yet waterproof.

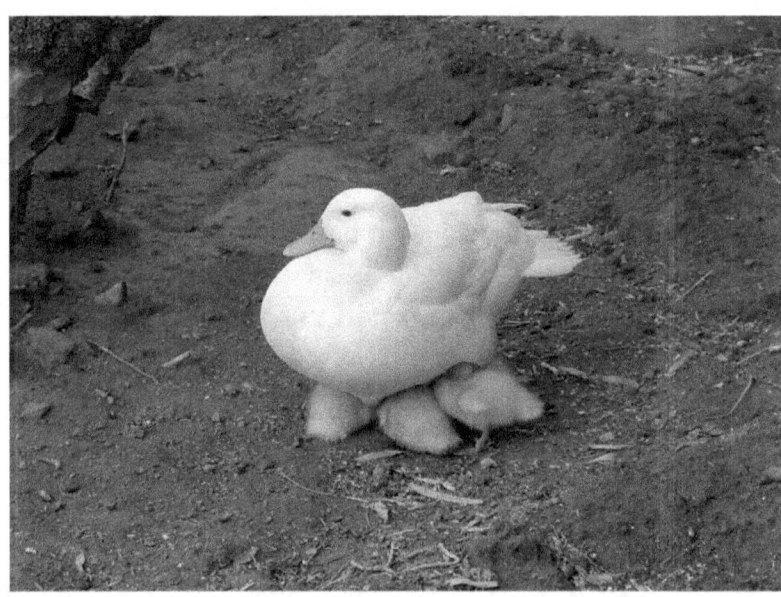

Keep the nest sawdust-free if you are using shavings, as this can block up the chicks digestive system and lead to an early demise!

Every predator likes a little duckling! So always keep the chicks protected from them. Be sure that rats cannot enter the area where they are kept, or you will lose the lot.

Be prepared with a heat lamp, just in case the mother abandons them early; this happens quite frequently so you must be prepared to give them a gentle source of heat to warm themselves – be careful not to cook them!

Ducklings grow pretty rapidly, and in a few short weeks they are perfectly well able to look after themselves – with a little help from you of course!

Feeding Time!

Ducks are great browsers, a bit like chickens except that they cannot scratch in the dirt as a hen does. However this does not inhibit them at all, and they love nothing better than to forage amongst leaf-litter or amongst foliage and weeds; even the vegetable patch – though admittedly they can do a bit of damage to your prize veggies if you are not careful.

They will happily hoover-up any slugs or insects that they find and will leave no stone unturned (literally) in their quest for grubs – I've even seen them gobble down a small mouse! If you have a pond or watercourse, then they will eat any small crustaceans or minnows they can find, as well as the young shoots of water plants.

When it comes to feeding them with 'store bought' food (which is **usually** essential to maintain a healthy diet); then free-range foraging Ducks only need fed once per day, while it is best to feed ducks in captivity twice daily. Give them as much to eat as they wish for about 15 minutes or so each time.

Commercial Pellets are usually best, but mash or corn, barley, oats etc helps balance the diet a little. Also, particularly Ducks that cannot forage will need a grit source nearby, to help with digestion and egg production. This is important as failure to provide a source of grit will lead to problems, sooner rather than later.

A little variety in the diet seems to be appreciated, and I still remember as a young lad mixing potatoes that had been boiled with their coats on, with oatmeal; for the Chickens, Geese and Turkeys that we kept – they absolutely loved it !

Water:

Ducks also need a clean regular water supply. This can be in the way of a pond, watercourse or just a tub of water to bathe in and drink from. Ducks need to be able to immerse their heads in water, in order to activate the preen valve under their tails and clean their feathers

This is an essential part of any water-fowls daily routine, and failure to supply clean water for their daily ablutions will result in unhealthy and unhappy birds!

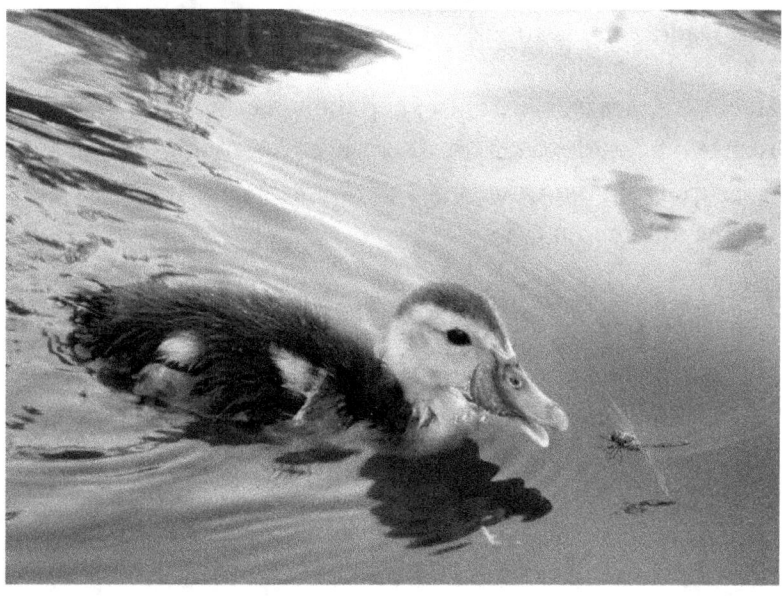

Indeed if you go anywhere near you're Ducks or Geese with a pail of water, they will immediately start quacking or honking excitedly if they have been neglected in this area. Put down the pail for a second – maybe while you are unlocking a gate – and they will undoubtedly try to get into it and spill the whole lot into the dirt!

Suspended waterers, where the duck cannot physically get into it and muck up the drinking water supply, as well as spill it over and mess up the bedding, are always best.

Nipple waterers are also a good idea – best to place them above a meshed area so that the water will seep away, and not be spread around the bedding material.

I must admit that it can be a bit of a challenge to keep an area that has Ducks in it clean – they love to splash in water and waddle in the muck!

Best I can advise here is to keep the watering area away from your residence if the ducks are free-range – and if you are supplying the water via a pail or other 'artificial' means, do keep it clean!

Foul water can lead to all sorts of disease and eye problems – in Ducks and humans alike.

Good Shelter

Like most farmyard poultry, good shelter is essential not just to keep the elements at bay; but also to protect your animals from the predations of hungry critters!

Ducklings in particular seem to be high on the list of favourable foods for hungry predators, from rats to foxes and raptors of all kinds. Hooded crows and rooks will soon fly away with any duckling they spot unprotected.

I have first-had experience in this aspect, when 12, 5-day old ducklings were stolen and stored behind a wall by rats. They left behind 12 chickens of exactly the same age, completely unscathed. Needless to say that it was the Rats last meal, as I hunted them down the very next day and removed the problem!

Special care has to be reserved for the miniatures, as even fully grown they can still be a tempting target for predators.

Housing

Housing your ducks depends very much on your own circumstances. For instance, if you are fortunate enough to have a decent sized pond, then this offers its own protection for the ducks during the day from dogs or foxes, and all you need is a shelter for them at night if necessary.

Most people however do not have this luxury, and so a decent sized shed must be provided, with a closed in area of 'open' ground attached where they can forage. Ducks do not roost as chickens do, but they will huddle together for warmth in colder weather. An area of around 2-3 square foot per duck is recommended in the shed.

Duck excreta contains 90% water, and so the bedding material must be changed regularly to avoid disease.

The bedding material can be straw, shavings, cut newspaper or even ground corncobs if you can get them. All are good, if they are dry and free from mould; although it is not recommended to use dusty shavings amongst ducklings under 7 days old as they will tend to eat the sawdust.

Be sure to regularly check the condition of your bedding, as Aspergillosis (caused by mould) can be devastating to your poultry if it is allowed to grow on the bedding material.

Adequate ventilation should also be provided, especially in the warm summer weather.

A nesting box should also be provided, although a constant watch must be taken with laying ducks, as some of them (like the Indian runner duck) will just drop their eggs where they stand!

A gently sloping ramp must be provided for them to enter and exit the shed without a struggle, which may damage their webbed feet.

Pen Perimeter Fence:

If you are badly troubled with strong predators such as fox or coyote, then you will need to keep your ducks in a secure enclosure.

This involves constructing a 'run' or enclosure with stout timbers and covered with a 2 inch galvanised or PVC covered weld mesh.

You might think that 2" weld mesh is a bit excessive but believe me a fox or Coyote can easily chew their way through the normal chicken wire – my own sister lost 5 of her chickens to a hungry fox by not taking this precaution!

The wire should be sunk into a trench around the perimeter to a depth of 12 inches or so, folding any slack towards the outside of the trench; and in turn should be covered with 1" galvanised chicken mesh then backfilled. This will keep out the smaller (but just as deadly) critters such as Stoats and Weasels.

2" Galvanise wire should cover the enclosure, and keep the fence height at around 6 foot, if you want to be able to walk in it without breaking your back in the process!

Duck Health

Ducks generally keep very good health and are fairly hardy creatures. However just like all living things, there are times when they need that bit of extra care due to accident or ill health.

Like most sickness, prevention is almost always better than cure, and as long as simple steps are taken to keep bedding and their environment clean and free from sharp obstacles, then with proper care and feed your ducks will keep good health.

There are some things that they can be prone to nevertheless, and it is always wise to know just what to do should you encounter health or other problems.

Here is a short list of the most common ailments, and what to do about them.

Aspergillosis:
The symptoms of Aspergillosis are laboured, heavy breathing, similar to pneumonia. This condition is usually caused by unclean, mouldy bedding material.

Treatment can involve fungicidal remedies, however good management regarding clean bedding and mould-free feed is the most effective long-term treatment.

Coccidiosis:

Symptoms usually start with blood in the droppings, followed by weak, thin birds, owing to the attack on the gut lining. Birds become very poorly for weeks.

Caused by birds foraging in ground infected by Coccidia, more common in hot wet conditions.
Treatment involves an anticoccidial medicine obtained from your vet, such as Harkers Coxoid.

Avoid future problems by grazing the young ducklings on clean grass and move the grazing area regularly so the ground does not become polluted/infected. As in all cases of this nature, clean food and water is essential for future prevention.

Botulism:

Symptoms of Botulism is a general loss of control in the neck, legs and wing movement; and an inability to swallow.
This is caused by allowing birds to graze amongst rotting vegetation and/or animal waste, resulting in bacterial infection.

Treated by firstly preventing birds from grazing in these conditions and also preventing swimming in any polluted water source.
Give the birds clean water to drink and seek advice of a vet for medication such as Epsom Salts & water.

Mites:

First symptoms of mites is excessive scratching; as the mites cause irritation by their blood-sucking activities. The causes of infection are often contact with other infected birds, or just from the ground where infected birds have been grazing.

Treatment is by pesticides (there are many to choose from). Always follow the instruction, especially with regard to withdrawal times for the treatment.

Maggots:

Symptoms for maggots – apart from the obvious – is a dirty, dry vent.

This is caused by too little water to drink or bathe in, especially during a hot summer.

Treatment involves picking away the maggots from the infected area, then treatment with a suitable spray or ointment (consult your vet), and of course making sure that the bird has enough clean water to prevent further problems.

Severe infestation can result in internal problems, and the bird having to be put down.

Sinus Problems:

Symptoms are puffed up cheeks and weeping nostrils, caused by bacteria.

Treatment is by an appropriate antibiotic injection from the vet. If left, this condition can lead to hardened cheeks and can become incurable.

Respiratory problems:

The symptoms of respiratory problems in your ducks is when they sit hunched-up and bob their tail up and down to assist in their breathing.
This is caused by a bacterial infection and is more common in very wet weather.
Treatment is by a course of antibiotic, supplied by your vet.

Worms:
Symptoms include a drop in egg production, accompanied by an increase in appetite.
Round and Tape worms can both be to blame, and can be picked up in the usual foraging activities – but especially on dirty infected ground.
Treatment involves a course of worming tablets obtained from your vet.

Lameness:
Symptoms of course is a limping duck! Lameness can be caused by many things, but special care has to be taken to be sure there are no sharp stones or other fragments in their area. Webbed feet can easily become split and infected, or legs damaged by careless handling.

If the cause is cut or infected feet, then appropriate treatment with ointment or antibiotics may be necessary. Isolate the infected duck for a few days on a bed of clean straw until the problem is resolved.

Disclaimer:
Even with this list of ailments and possible solutions to hand, it is always recommended to consult your local animal doctor or vet, if in any doubt at all. This list of

possible ailments/diseases is intended as a general guide only, and not intended as veterinary advice.

Preparing For The Table

If you are keeping your ducks for eggs only, or even for pets, then this section may not interest you. However the fact is that many will keep Ducks for meat and eggs, so a knowledge of how to humanly slaughter then dress your Duck is essential in this respect.

First rule when keeping any animal that you may wish to slaughter at a later date – and this is especially for the kids - **Do not name it!** Names are for friends, and unless your name is Hannibal Lecter, you do not eat your friends!

I was always brought up on the principle that where there is livestock – there is dead stock (my father's words of wisdom). A working farm or homesteading has no 'pets' (well maybe one or two) and death is all a part of the process of living.

Preparing any animal for your own use and preparing it for commercial sale is a different matter entirely; with commercial preparation involving the proper permits and compliance with local regulation. If you are preparing birds for sale to the public, then you must seek the proper advice from your local authority to do so.

Ducks For Eggs:

Bearing in mind that even though a duck may be kept for its egg production – it may well end up on the table! There are some things that you should know when it comes to keeping ducks for eggs rather than primarily for their meat.

First thing is that a duck will start to produce eggs around 4-5 months old, similar to a chicken. The laying time however is considerably longer than the average chicken, which tends to fade away at 2-3 years.

A good laying duck such as the Buff Orpington for instance, will go on to lay for up to 5 or 6 years no problem, although with age there is a gradual decrease in egg numbers. It is generally thought that keeping your ducks 'Drake free' will increase the overall egg yield.

So with that said, let's get on with the business of slaughtering and preparing your duck for the kitchen table.

Slaughtering:

The best age to slaughter a duck is a matter of some debate, as larger ducks such as the Rouen, can be considered big enough at 8-12 weeks, whilst smaller species like the Khaki Campbell can be as late as 16-20 weeks.
The basic rule of thumb though is that the younger the birds, then the more tender the meat.

Other things to consider is the amount of feed they will consume over the longer period vs the advantages of the larger carcase; also the fact that the pin feathers can be a real challenge to remove in the older birds.

Before slaughter it is always best to let the duck fast for a period of 12 hours or so, with access to water only. This gives time for the crop to empty and reduces the risk of contamination when dressing the animal.

When it comes to actually killing the bird, then it is essential that this is done as humanely as possible and that the animal does not suffer needlessly.

There are many methods of dispatching the bird, but this is one that I find the most effective.
Either tie the birds wings together with twine, or place in a canvas bag leaving only the head and neck protruding; this is just to prevent the wings flapping around.

Gripping the bird firmly by the legs, Lay the birds neck under a broom handle laid on a frim floor, with your feet on either side; and with a sharp tug, pull upwards.

Alternatively stamp down hard on the broom with one foot to break the neck – be sure that it is set on firm ground though, so that the neck is properly broken and not just crushed.

These methods will break the neck and lead to instant death – be careful not to pull too harshly otherwise the head may come off entirely, which is rather messy to say the least!
Place the bird upside down in a bleeding cone (an old road cone with the top cut off will do fine), and slit the throat to bleed the bird.

Plucking:
Apart from hot waxing, which involves dunking your fully feathered duck into a hot bath of water and melted wax – then removing the down feathers after they have coated and cooled on the bird - there are two traditional ways to pluck fowl by hand, dry plucking and wet plucking.

The dry plucking method is simply to pull the feathers from the bird while it is still warm. Starting with the heavy wing feathers and tail feathers, which you will sharply pull straight out.

The body feathers are removed by holding the bird firmly and pulling the feathers 'against the grain' being careful not to tear the bird in the process.

This generally results in a cleaner more attractive carcase; the downside is that it is also easier to tear the skin and is a harder job overall than wet plucking.

The wet plucking method involves heating up a barrel of water to around 60C and dunking the bird into it by the feet for a few minutes.

This makes the feathers much easier to remove, with less chance of tearing the flesh. It can however lead to some flesh discoloration, especially if the bird is dunked for too long.

Sometimes it is impossible to remove the pin hairs on the bird, and so a light going-over with a small blowtorch can be used to remove them.

If the feathers are being kept for duvet or pillow stuffing, then this is the time to separate the down and small body feathers from the large wing and tail feathers. The down can be used for the duvet, and the small body feathers for stuffing pillows and the like.

Both should be washed in a gentle detergent; thereafter scattered on a surface covered in a soft, porous material in a suitable room to dry out – or sealed into pillow cases and placed in a tumble dryer.

Evisceration:

Simply insert the knife into the vent at the rear and slit the flesh to the breastbone. Insert your hand high up into the body cavity and pull back to remove the internal organs. Remove the head and cut off the legs at the hock joints.

Wash the bird thoroughly inside and out. If the giblets are to be kept, then wash thoroughly and place into a suitable plastic bag. Place inside the carcase, or keep separate.

Freshly killed birds should be dressed as soon as possible, thereafter stored in a fridge for use within 5-7 days.

Popular Domestic Duck Breeds

Indian Runner Duck

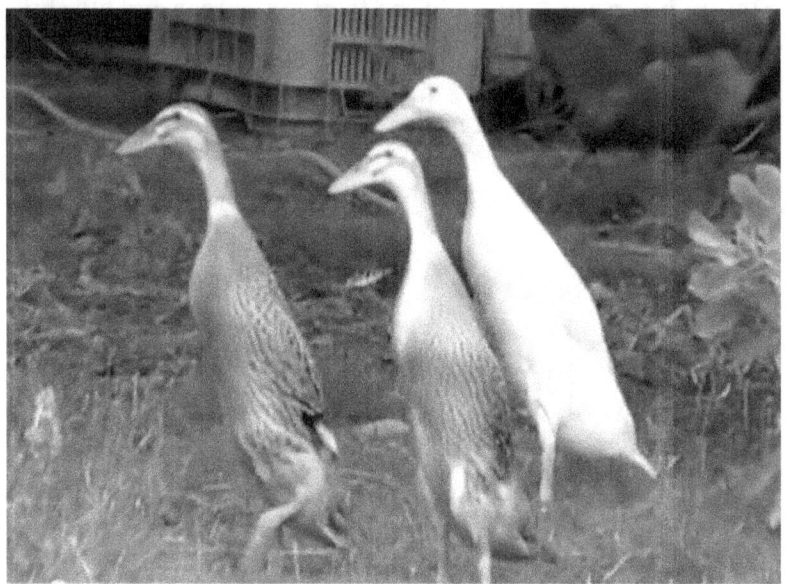

This is perhaps familiar to many people as the star in the 'Babe' movies! A hugely popular duck with its distinctive long neck and its general upright posture - giving it a real mischievous look.

These ducks come in a variety of colours, and like all ducks, they love water, but are most happy foraging amongst leaf litter and vegetation.

This duck is often in demand to train sheep dogs, when there are no sheep available, owing to its propensity to flock together and be guided; they run rather than waddle.

They can lay over 250 eggs per year, and drop them wherever they stand, so duck breeders have to keep a good watch over them if they are not to lose the eggs to predators!

American Pekin Duck

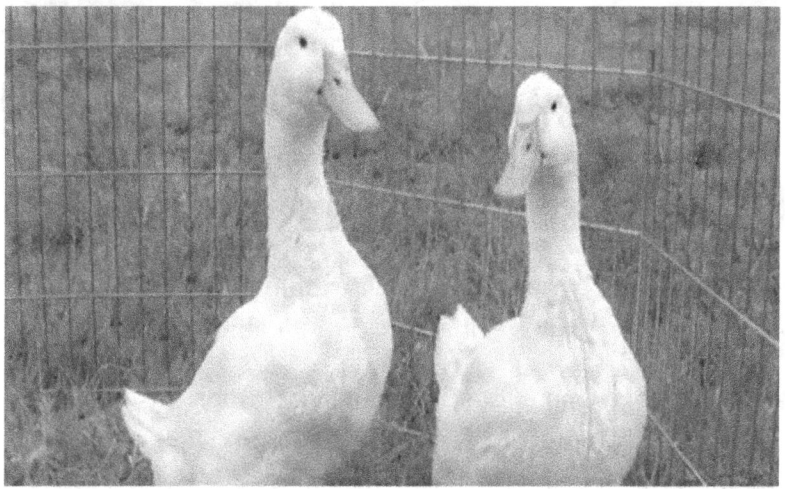

Originally bred from the Mallard duck in China, the Pekin or Long Island Duck, has gone on to become the favourite of the domestic ducks in the United States today, accounting for over 95% of all the duck meat consumed.

Crested Pekin:

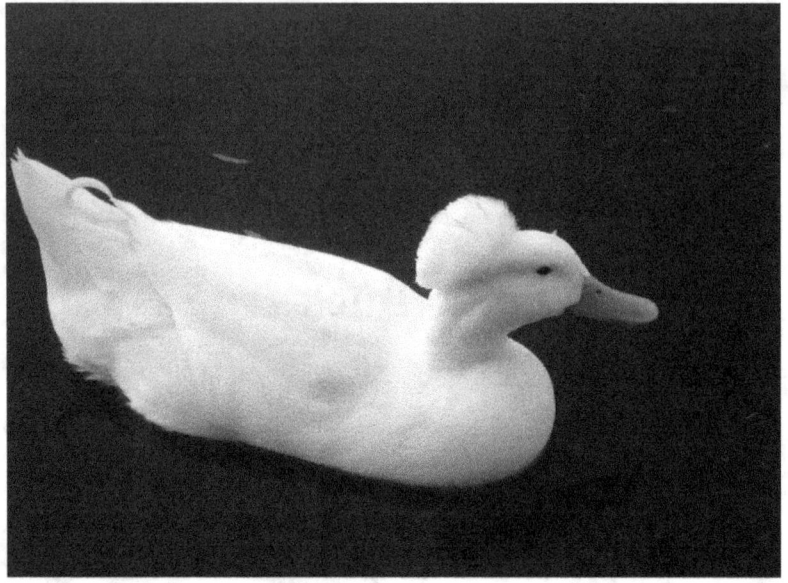

It is also a fairly good layer, and can lay over 200 eggs per year - as long as it is not allowed to incubate them.

If however you intend to hatch the eggs, then it is best to use a broody hen for the purpose, as Pekin Ducks will commonly abandon the nest before the eggs are hatched.

As one of the more intelligent species, they also make good companions or pets, and easily bond with other animals and humans, making them a favourite with the kids!

Khaki Campbell

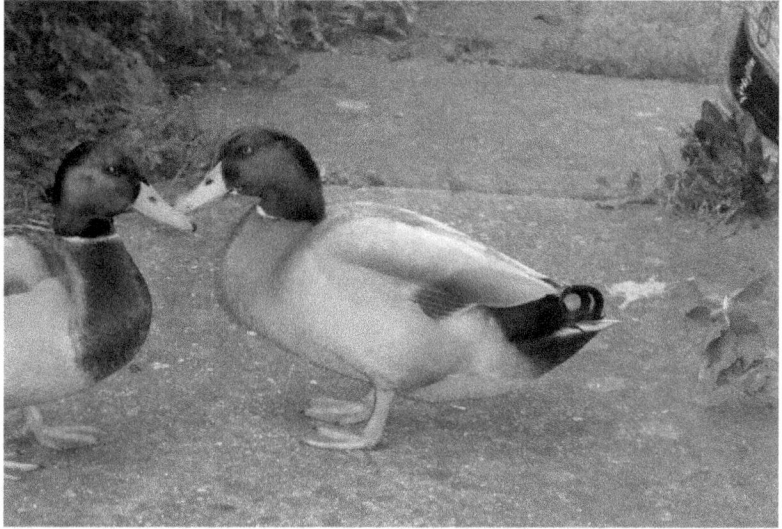

A cross between the Mallard, Rouen and Runner ducks, the Khaki Campbell originated in England at the turn of the 19th century.

Weighing in at 3 – 5lbs, it is not the largest of breeds, but is a prolific egg-layer managing around 320 tasty eggs per year; this puts it on a par with even the best laying chickens.

It is this egg-laying ability that makes up for the fact that they are not the best of brooders, and often an incubator or broody hen is best for hatching the eggs – which takes between 23-28 days.

Rouen Duck

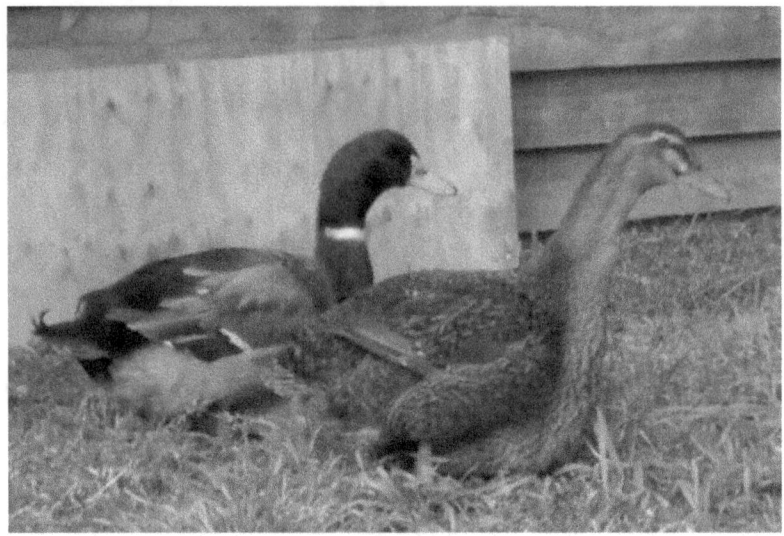

The Rouen drake and hen are almost identical in appearance to the Mallard, the only real distinguishing factor being that the Rouen is slightly larger and the colouring bolder.

This is a Duck bred mainly for the meat, as it weighs in at a healthy 9-12lbs; whilst the egg production is only between 30-120 eggs per year.

Of French extraction, and introduced to the USA in 1850; the flesh of the Rouen is dark but full of flavour.

Muscovy

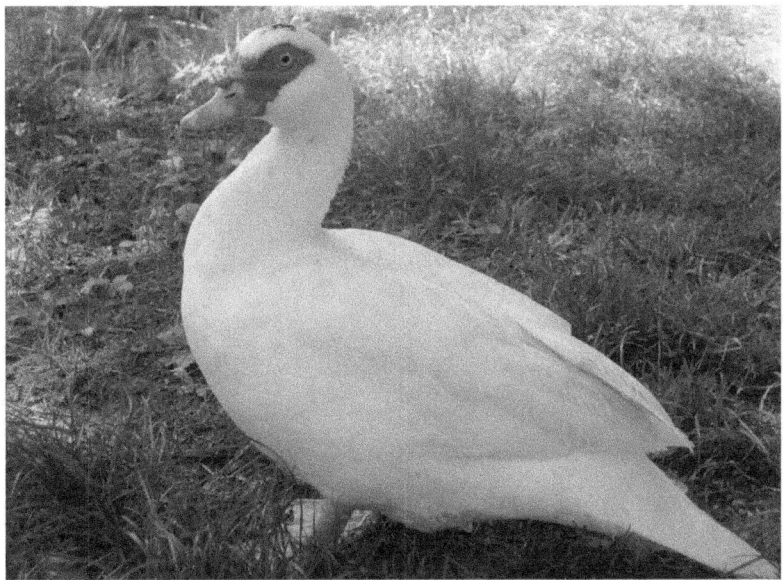

The only breed of ducks that is not descended from the Mallard; this is a popular duck amongst those that like their meat dark and strong flavoured.

It is also leaner with less fat than the Mallard-derived breeds and is often compared to veal or roast beef! The male can grow to an impressive 15lbs, the female generally being half that size.

Frequently cross-bred with Mallards, resulting in a 'Mullard' duck, that is generally accepted as 'kosher' amongst the Jewish community.

This duck is popular where there are neighbours nearby, as it is also known as a 'quack-less' duck in that it is very quiet as it goes about its business. They come in a variety of colours, but black & White or white only, are the most predominant.

Buff Orpington

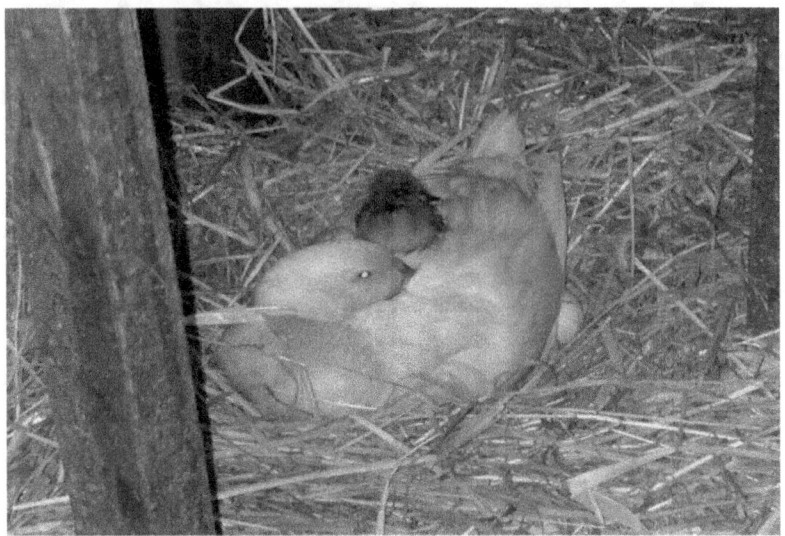

Getting its name from Orpington in Kent; where it was originally bred by William Cook in the early 1900's, this is a prolific egg-layer laying over 220 eggs per year, but is also very popular for its meat, being a medium weight bird of around 7 to 8 lbs.

The fact that its light pin feathers do not show up on the plucked carcase, is another thing that endears this duck to breeders rearing it for meat.

Regarded as being one of the most attractive of ducks, it has nevertheless been in decline over recent years.

Bantam Duck Breeds

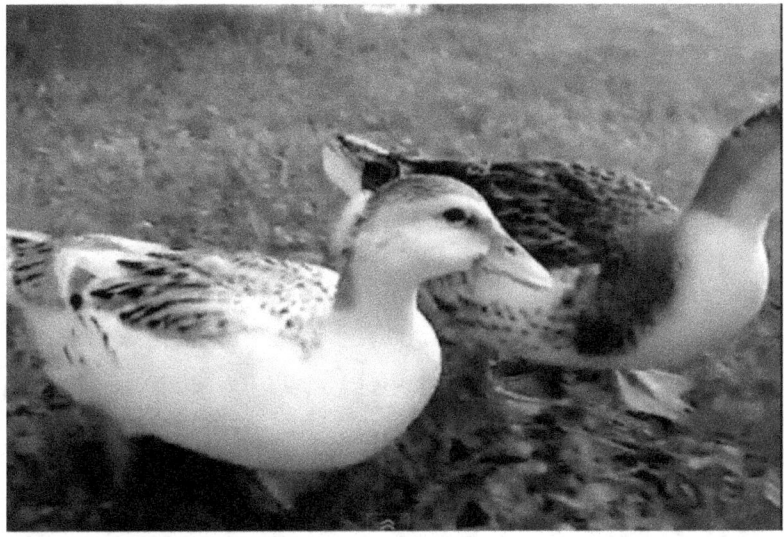

Bantam ducks are also known as miniatures, or generically 'call ducks' owing to the fact that this small duck was originally bred to lure in ducks to the guns by their loud quacks.

They are generally between ¼ to 1/3 the size of their larger strains. Not generally reared for their meat (there are exceptions), they are however often reared for their eggs, and indeed as pets for the kids!

If ascetics are what you are looking for, or a little living decoration for your homestead, then these little ducks make an absolutely charming back-drop – as well as making only a fraction of the mess that a traditional duck will make.

One of the downsides however is that they tend to be a little flighty, so sometimes need their wings clipped. They are also a big attraction for foxes and other predators including Buzzards or kites, that can easily carry them off.

Even though they are regarded as ornamental, they do have some real attributes including the fact that they can make good sitters, and they love to forage amongst the vegetation thereby keeping tight control over the usual garden pests.

I have found that the children quickly take to these charming creatures, and so it is a good way to introduce the kids to the craft involved in caring for a vulnerable living creature – a skill that will last a lifetime.

Silver Appleyard Miniature

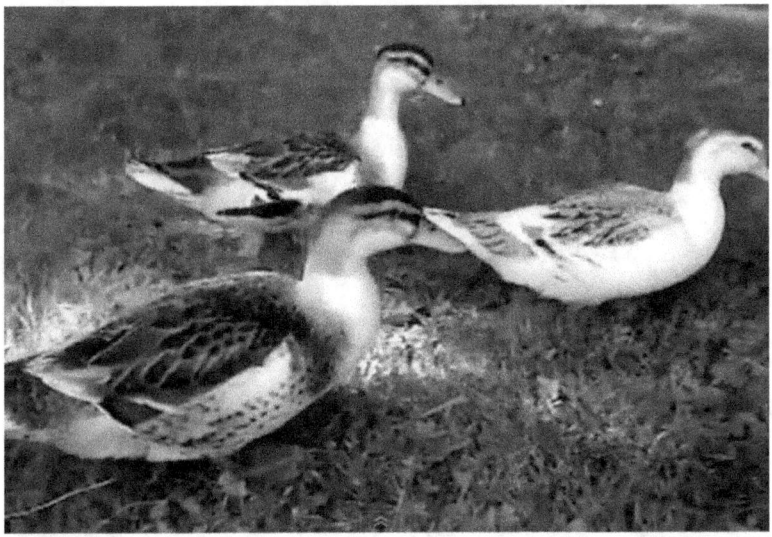

The Silver Appleyard is perhaps one of the most popular of the bantam breeds. Very friendly and sociable, they will chatter constantly when excited – or a suitable water bath is offered!

Not prolific egg-layers, they produce a white to olive green egg. They also make great setters and are one of the hardiest of the Bantam Duck breeds.

East Indie Bantam

This attractive miniature is well favoured by those seeking to exhibit their birds. The striking black sheen makes this miniature stand out in the crowd so to speak, and the fact that they are a little quieter than call ducks is an added bonus!

They do make good flyers, so they must be kept clipped or in a closed environment be it cage or run.

Traditional Call Duck

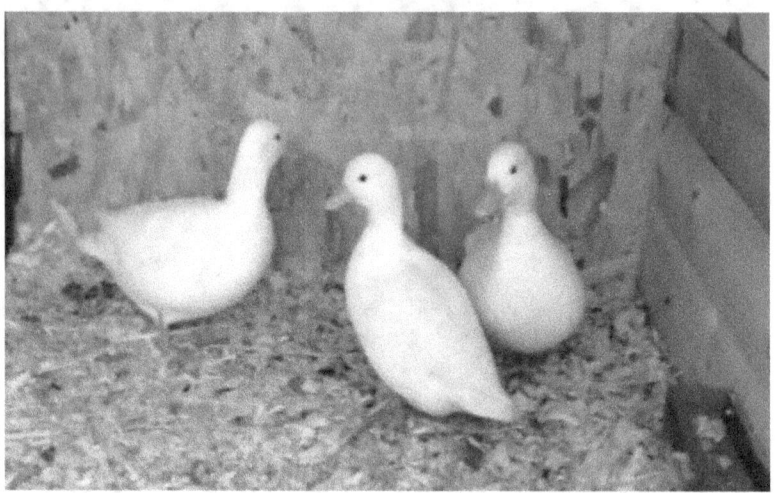

As mentioned earlier, the Call Duck is sometimes used in a general sense for all of the miniature breeds. However the true nature of the Call duck was to do just that – Call.

This is a small duck especially bred for its loud quack by hunters, to lure in their bigger cousins.

They make great entertainment as they noisily go about their foraging, and the kids love them!

Title 2 - Gourmet Geese!

Homesteading Animals (3): Gourmet Geese!

Rearing Geese For Meat, Eggs & Feather Pillows!

By
Norman J Stone

www.deanburnpublications.com

Introduction

I was brought up in a homestead environment, where I was in charge of the poultry on our small steading from a young age. The lessons I learned (even though I did not appreciate them at the time!) over this period have stood me in good stead over the years, and I have never regretted the time spent cleaning out and caring for the animals in my charge; whilst my friends were away playing football and having a great time…well, maybe just a little!

The fact is that caring for animals does eat up a lot of your time, it is just the way it is. However with proper organization or routine, it does not necessarily have to eat away your 'me' time altogether. Poultry in particular does not have to massively time consuming, and the rewards in terms of meat or eggs produced, far outweigh the work or time involved in its production.

The self-sustainable lifestyle is all about working for your own (including your families) benefit; for financial, material, even mental gain – for there is nothing quite as satisfying as enjoying the fruits of your labour whether it be in the form of meat, eggs, fruit or vegetables.

With all that understood, this book is all about one of the most popular Christmas birds throughout American and Europe especially – the domestic Goose; the most popular Christmas bird at the moment of course is the Turkey (Book coming soon!). This was not always the case however, and in the 18-19th century, Goose was very much the Christmas favourite.

Both of these fantastic birds are raised primarily for their meat, or even for security; however they can and do produce large tasty eggs – especially in the case of the Chinese Goose which can lay around 30-45 eggs per year.

I hope that you will enjoy this introduction to keeping Geese, and if you are not doing so already, will seriously consider rearing Geese for yourself and enjoying the many benefits to be had.

***

Beginning With Geese

I began my poultry career with a flock of a dozen or so Chinese Geese, raised from goslings that my father bought at the local poultry market. They were a great introduction to caring for animals, and along with a selection of Ducks, kept me constantly busy and entertained!

Geese are grazing animals, and we were fortunate enough to have a large old orchard that had plenty of grass between the trees, and made an ideal foraging for these active birds.

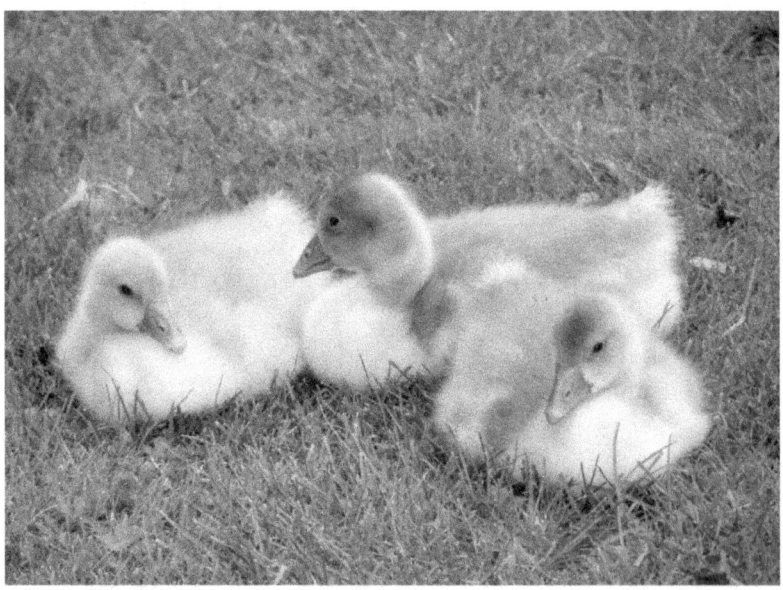

They in turn warned us as soon as any strangers came near; day or night they make an ideal early warning system – better than any electronic alarm!

In fact Geese are used for security by many business owners, from jailhouses in Brazil, to distilleries in

Scotland. As they are light sleepers, they are almost impossible to sneak past any time of day or night, and even just a couple of Geese will put up the most piercing din if alarmed by a stranger.

They can also be quite intimidating when you are not used to them, and I well remember my friend coming to visit me one day as I was about to go and feed my flock.

They were grazing at the top of our long orchard which sloped uphill, and when I called them with my usual 'come and get it!' they all took off running towards me, finally lifting of the ground and breaking into a short flight.

The effect was quite dramatic, as they headed in a broad line straight towards us. I of course was used to such behaviour and new they would suddenly settle to ground right in front of me; my friend however knew no such thing, and when I turned to speak to him – he was off running terrified in the opposite direction.

Of course I thought it was hilarious, and ribbed him about it for weeks - Ah….Happy days!

They are also ideal for many business owners that have an abundance of open grass to cut, as a small flock of 5 or so Geese will happily munch away about 1 full acre of grassland - leaving less grass for the mowers to cut down.

Yes, they do need cared for; as does any living thing. However they are hardy creatures, and provided they have adequate food, water and shelter; then they really are little trouble at all, and in many ways can be a real advantage to have around.

In fact, if you have the space to keep these wonderful birds, then here is a short-list of 6 good reasons why you should consider keeping Geese on your Homesteading or farm area.

1: Meat

Geese are a great source of nutritious tasty meat, with a full-grown domestic Goose such as the Emden growing up to a massive 34lbs! This can be a major contributor to the family food intake.

2: Eggs

Some goose varieties such as the White Chinese can produce over 60 rich tasty eggs per year. Calculate 1 goose egg to equal 2-3 large hens eggs and try out your favourite recipes with them – you may be in for a pleasant surprise!

3: Security

As mentioned earlier; geese make great 'guard dogs.' Ideal security around the farm or homestead, they will surely let you know if there are any intruders about – animal or human!

4: Living Mowers!

If you have a large area of grass that you need mowed constantly, and it is fenced in to stop the geese wandering off, then consider keeping geese instead of a motorized grass cutting machine. They'll happily munch away at the grass – and they're better to look at.

5: Goose Down

The small fluffy feathers under the belly of the Goose are where Goose Down comes from. This can be used to stuff your goose-down bed throw, and the smaller Goose feathers to stuff your cosy feather pillows!

6: Company!
Yes, geese make great companions, and will easily bond with the person who feeds them. Their antics can keep you amused for ages – especially around feeding or watering time.

Geese can live for over 30 years – so you can appreciate them for longer than the family dog or cat!

Be aware though…if you intend to eat them later – Do Not Name them. It's fairly straight-forward to kill and eat an animal; but it's not natural at all to eat your friend!

***

Popular Breeds

Emden (or Embden)

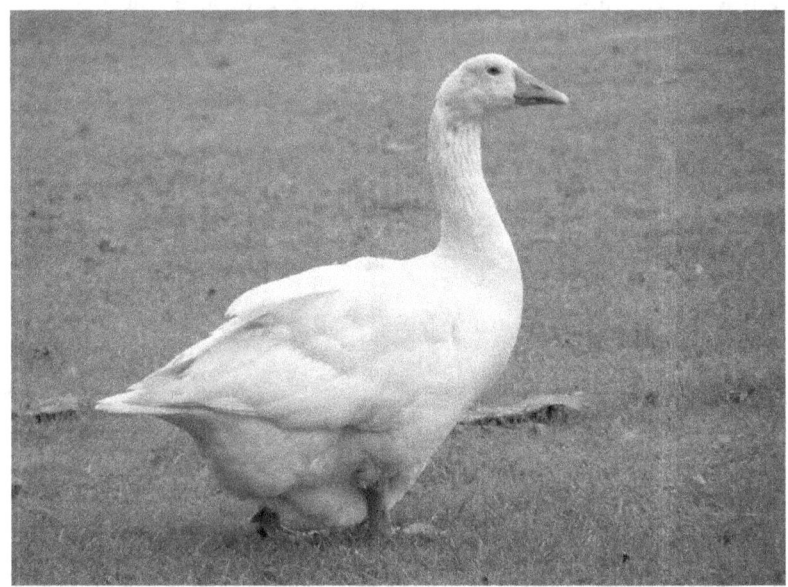

All white with an orange beak and blue eyes, this is a very popular and fast-growing Goose, quickly reaching 20lbs and more.

The Emden is a white breed with orange beak and feet.

Maturing at 2-3 years, it is a strong bird and is often used as a guard 'dog' owing to its willingness to defend its territory from strangers.

Laying around 35 or so eggs per year and almost twice the size of other domestic Geese, guarantees the Emden a high ranking amongst Homesteaders and hobby farmers alike. They are good parents and will often raise a full nest of Goslings with no problems at all.

Brecon Buff

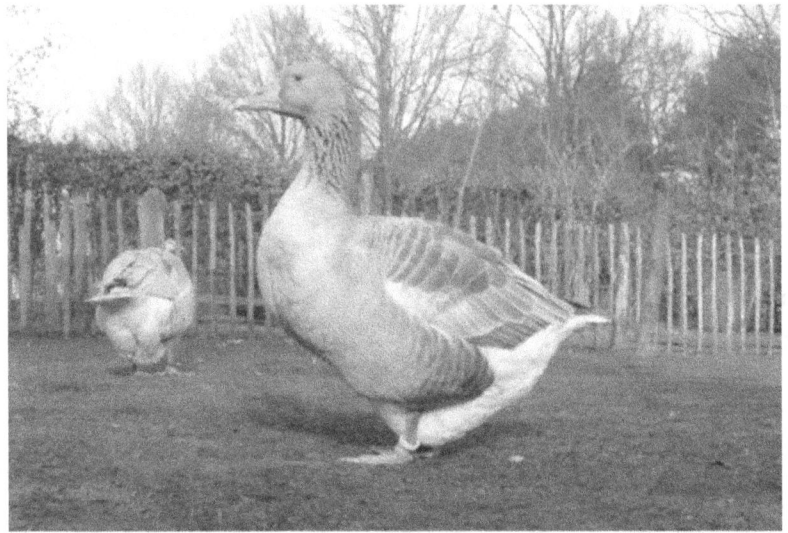

If you are looking for a Goose to show, then this one would make a good choice. Definitely one of the most attractive of breeds, the Brecon Buff is a hardy animal and able to stand harsh weather quite comfortably.

They make very good parents and are traditionally reared for the Christmas table. Originating from the Brecon Beacons in Wales, they are a medium-weight bird and need a good supply of grazing to grow to full weight of around 8kg (17lbs 10 0z).

One of the rarer breeds of Goose.

White Chinese

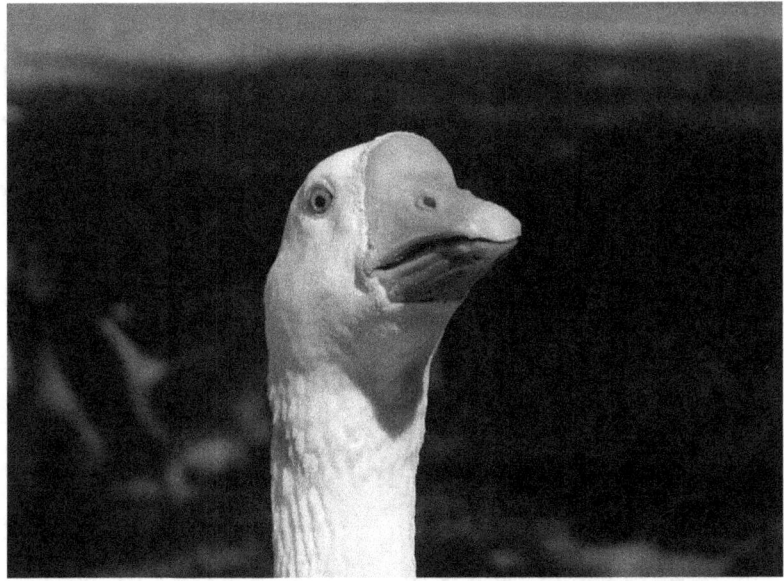

This is definitely one of the most popular 'guard geese' amongst breeders, owing to it being just that bit more inquisitive and noisy than the other breeds.

Colours range between pure white, grey and brown, and it has a distinctive knob at the top of its beak.

This is a good choice if Goose eggs are your target, as the Chinese can lay over 60 eggs per year; making them one of the top egg-layers in the Goose family.

Weighing in at around 22lbs for a mature male, this is one of the larger breeds and so is ideal also for meat production. Care has to be taken over the winter periods that the knob on the beak does not get damaged by hard frosty weather.

African Goose

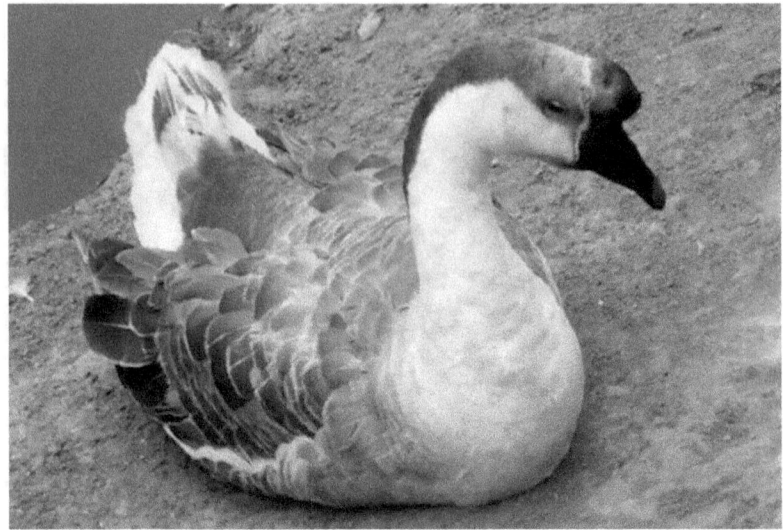

The African is an example of perhaps the largest of the domestic Geese, weighing at around 22lbs for the Gander and 18 lbs for the Goose, it is not African at all, but actually a descendant of the wild Swan Goose.

It is again subject to damage to the knob at the beak by frost, so care has to be taken to protect it in bad weather.

Not a big layer, it nevertheless can produce around 40 large white eggs over the season. A long-lived bird, It has a distinctive dewlap that hangs from its upper jaw and lower neck.

Pilgrim

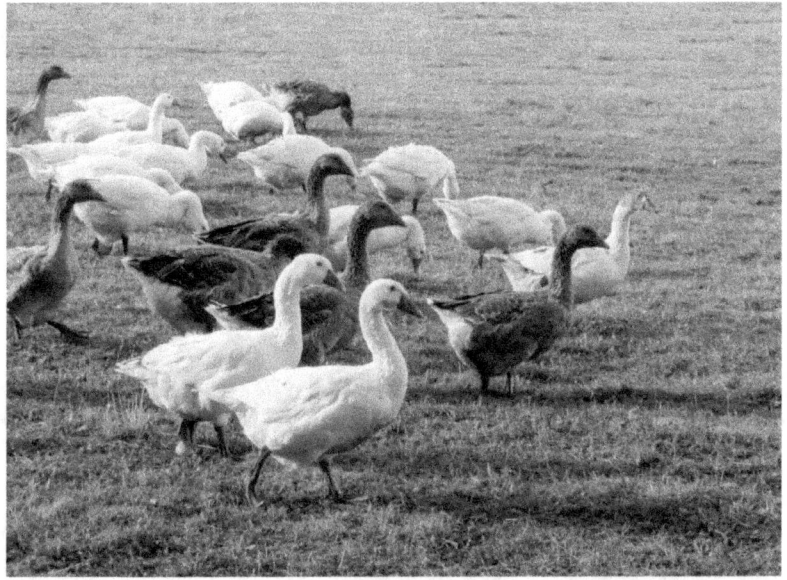

This is an example of an auto-sexing Goose, where the sex can easily be determined by the colour. In the case of the Pilgrim, the Gander is all-white while the Goose is a medium grey.

Thought to be descended from another auto-sexing breed – the West of England Goose – this bird is one of only two American auto-sexing breeds (the other being the Cotton Patch breed).

It is a medium-sized Goose, the Gander reaching about 14lbs at maturity. Producing around 40 eggs during the season, it particularly enjoys ranging, and is known to be a docile breed to work with.

This, and the fact that it is easy to tell the males from the females, makes them an ideal breed for beginners

Toulouse

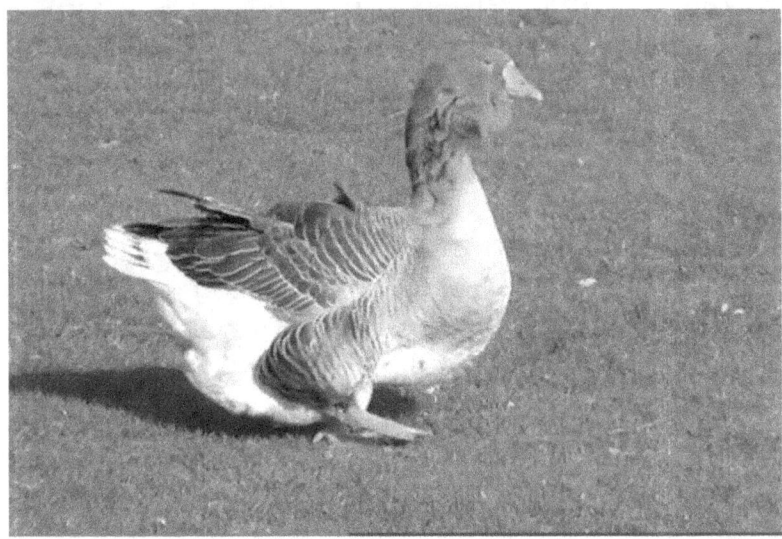

This breed was initially developed for its large liver, from which was made the famous 'pate de foie gras.' A very large bird, they do not need a large area as they are not keen to forage.

Also the fact that they have very large feet, means that they can make a fair mess of poorly drained land.

A popular show bird, it can also lay around 35 eggs per year, though mostly they are reared for show or for their meat (the full grown Gander can reach an impressive 30lbs).

Not recommended as a bird for beginners as they are prone to things such as fly strike, where flies lay eggs on their feathers particularly around the vent area, resulting in maggot infestation if not properly treated.

There are two breeds of this magnificent bird, the Grey Toulouse and the Buff variety. They also have good soft feathering, and so are often used for Goose-down production.

Roman

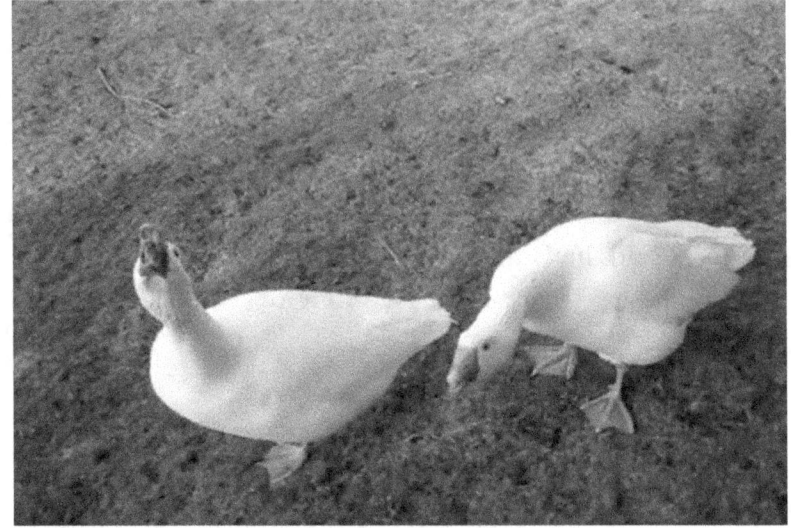

Originating in Italy over 2,000 years ago, this bird is also known as the 'Crested Roman' owing to the small crest shaped like a tiny helmet on its head. Predominantly reared as a small roasting bird – it only reaches around 12lbs – it also produces around 35 eggs per year.

Known to be alert and sociable, it is an ideal beginner's bird that is fairly hardy and easily cared for. They make ideal 'watch dogs' and will soon alert you to the presence of strangers or predators.

To Summarise:

- Decide whether your priorities are meat or eggs – or even downy feathers, before choosing your bird.

- If you are attempting to breed pure-breds, then purchase from a reputable dealer
- Consider the breed type and temperament – will it suit the kids?
- How much free grazing do you have? Choose your bird accordingly for little or lots of grazing land.
- If you are considering a noisy Goose, then think of the neighbours and the possible complaints!
- If you are a beginner to rearing Geese, then consider a smaller bird such as the Roman – then perhaps progress to the larger breeds when ready for them.
- When first releasing your Geese, keep pet dogs and noisy children away from them, and gradually introduce them to their environment.

***

Caring For Geese

Shelter:

When it comes to building a shelter for your Geese, it does not have to be anything that will win Best Construction or design awards! The fact is that Geese are great grazers, and much prefer to roam around foraging for food – or even just out of sheer inquisitiveness.

Inclement Weather does not trouble them much at all, unless it is severe indeed. With this in mind then your shelter has to do two things in the main; and that is to protect them from predators and the weather when it is really bad.

Predators are perhaps your biggest concern, for even large Geese such as the Emden or African, will not be able to fend off a determined attack from a fox or stray dog.

With this in mind, it may be necessary to herd them into a secure shelter in the evening. Either that or enclose the whole area with a high predator proof fence, and leave the shelter open for them to gain access when they need it.

The shelter can take the form of a garden shed or a small barn. As long as it is weather and predator proof and allows about 1 square yard floor space for every bird. Overcrowding will only lead to respiratory and other problems. It should also be well ventilated (not draughty).

The floor of the shelter should be covered in straw, sand or shavings; and should be cleaned out regularly. Perhaps a deep clean once per week, and a general going-over daily – depending on conditions.

***

Pasture & Feed:

Geese love to graze, perhaps with the exception of the Toulouse which likes to stay near water and the food trough! However in general Geese are great foragers and will travel a fair distance grazing constantly.

This of course means that to keep happy geese, then you must have adequate grazing for them. A good rule of thumb is to have 1 acre of grass to about 5 or 6 geese, depending on the quality and abundance of this resource. Bear in mind also that grass grows fastest over the spring period and so calculations will vary over the course of the year.

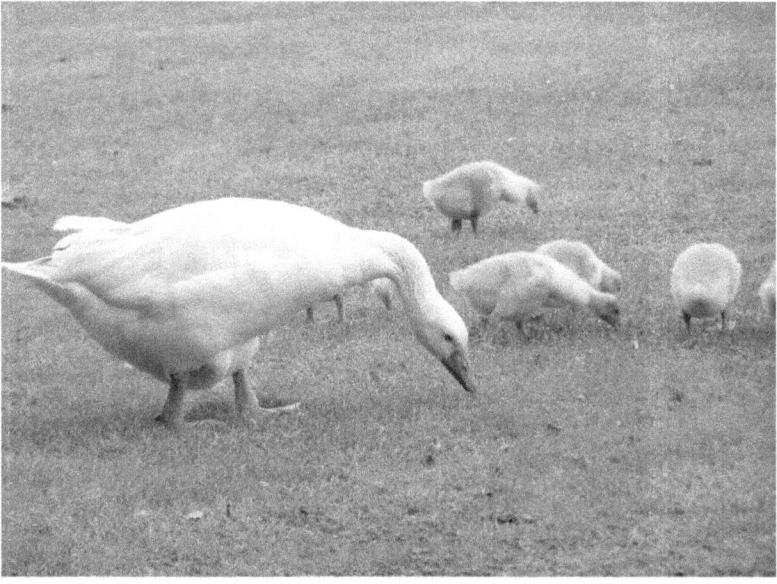

It is usually the case that as the grass grows sparse then artificial feed must be introduced in the form of manufactured pellets or mash. This will be adapted according to the growth stage of your stock, as Goslings are best fed on a starter pellet and older birds on a maintenance pellet to supplement their diet of grass during lean times, or if the grass is poor quality.

Geese will also happily munch away on any left-over vegetable cuttings from the kitchen, or thinning's from the veggie patch. For a special treat I have fed mine watermelon – and they love it! Also try a little peanut butter on a slice of brown bread, feed by hand and win a friend for life ☺ Apples and other fruit is usually appreciated.

Before letting your birds out to graze, be sure to check for poisonous plants such as Laburnum, Deadly Nightshade or Yew. Also check for any foreign objects that may cause damage to their webbed feet, or indeed if they are ingested by the bird.

Old bits of barbed wire fencing, or baling twine can cause terrible damage to your flock, and a rusty nail up the foot does nobody any good!

Always make sure there is adequate clean water available. This is important not only for their digestive system, but also to enable them to clean up properly as it is by constant preening that they are able to keep themselves weather-proof.

Dipping their heads up to the neck in clean water also helps to clean their eyes and nostrils out properly, preventing the onslaught of infection.

Finally, make sure that there is an adequate source of grit available for your Geese. All fowl need grit to aid in their digestion, as the grit works in the crop to break down the food and aid in their digestion.

If they are free-range, then this is not usually a problem as they will pick up an abundance of grit during their foraging. If kept indoors for any length of time though, be sure to have a grit-bin within easy reach.

***

Gosling Care:

Geese are monogamous creatures and will mate for life. During the nesting season a goose will sit on 2 – 9 eggs for a period of 24-28 days. The incubation period starts from the last egg laid, and after she starts to sit on the nest.

Upon hatching the Goslings are immediately mobile and able to begin foraging for their food.

Always have a heat lamp prepared, just in case the parent abandons the chicks. Like humans, some make better mothers than others! Particularly in new mums this may happen to Goslings; however a simple heat lamp on a string above an area indoors will be enough to give them the extra heat they need.

Make sure it is a minimum 2 feet above the ground, and that the chicks can move away from it if it is too hot. As they get older and get feathers, gradually replace with a normal 100-watt lamp before weaning them off it entirely.

Make sure Goslings under two weeks or so, do not have access to deep water, as their downy coats are not fully water-resistant, and they may well freeze or drown.

During this time the parents, particularly the Gander is likely to show aggressive behaviour such as hissing or flapping wings, to anyone who approaches the chicks. This is perfectly natural behaviour and will help keep away predators – just watch out for the kids!

Goslings are not much trouble at all, especially if you have two caring parents to watch over them. There are however a few things that you should watch out for regarding their general health and well-being.

For the first couple of weeks or so, the small birds are in danger from any number of predators, from stoats and rats to the larger badgers, foxes, stray dogs and every other carnivore out there; the variety and numbers will only vary according to your particular location.

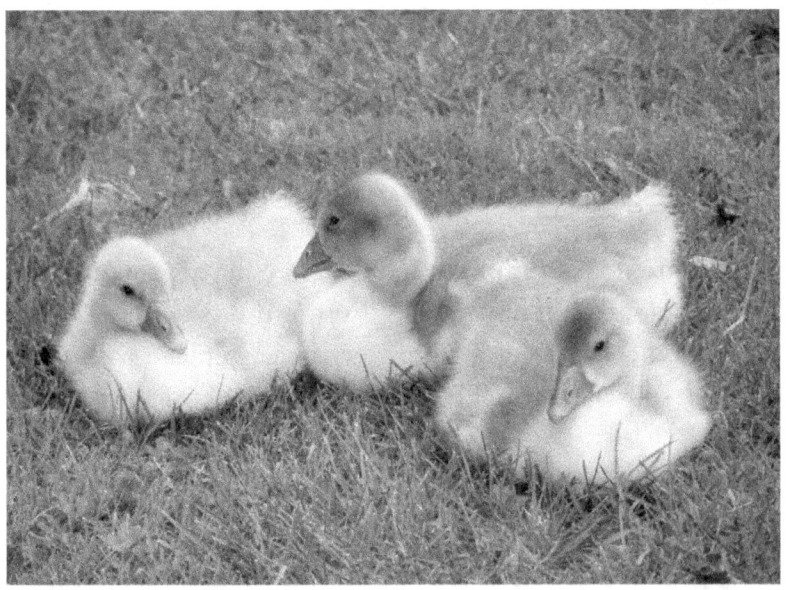

As well as the four-legged predators there are also the raptors to watch out for, and you may well have to keep your Goslings under cover for at least 3-4 weeks if you have any Red Kites or larger raptors in the skies above you.

Larger Goose breeds such as the African or Emden with their huge feet, can also crush new chicks; so be sure that the chicks have plenty of room (especially if they are housed indoors) to get out of the way.

Goslings are however very fast growers, and within a few weeks will soon be out of most danger – apart from the larger predators of course.

Be sure also that you do not use powdery wood shavings as bedding when the goslings are first born, as they will ingest the sawdust and likely perish as a result.

With regard to manufactured feed stuffs. Do not feed them dry mash (even mixed as it should be with water) for the first 2 weeks or so, as this is likely to choke them. Also be aware that too much high protein may result in 'wing droop.'

This is because their muscles have not developed fast enough to keep up with their body mass. For this reason if feed is required be sure that it is suitable for the young birds, and is not too protein-rich.

Allowing the Goslings room to play and flap their wings, helps with muscle development and will go a long way to producing healthy young adults.

***

Keeping Healthy Geese

Most breeds of domestic Geese are fairly hardy creatures and if fed well and kept in clean conditions, they will not easily succumb to illness or disease. With that said however, there are a few things to watch out for in order for your Geese to remain in good health.

Issues regarding sharp objects and other contaminants that may injure them if they are stood on or ingested, were covered in one of the previous chapters; so there is no need to repeat that here.

However there are a number of other things that can lead to an unhappy (or dead!) bird – here is a list of some of the most common of them, with their symptoms and treatments.

Fowl Cholera:

Also known as Pasteurellosis, this is a highly contagious disease and should be treated immediately – the bird also being quarantined. Fowl Cholera usually appears as a septicaemic disease and is so fast moving that sometimes death is the first sign of its presence!

It is mostly caused by infection through poor sanitary practices, and so the first step in the treatment is to clean up the living environment – particularly any contaminated water supply – and isolate any infected birds.

The Vet should be called upon to properly diagnose and treat the bird, and vaccinate the rest of the flock to prevent further infection.

Aspergillosis:

Aspergillosis is defined as any disease condition caused by a member of the fungal genus Aspergillus. It is a fungal disease that infects the lungs and can even infect the embryo in the egg.

Again this is usually a result of poor hygiene management, resulting in dirty infected eggs that can infect both the sitter and the unborn chick.

Symptoms involve heavy laboured breathing, with gasping gurgling or other noises from the infected bird. General lethargy and poor appetite will accompany these symptoms.

Prevention as usual is better than the cure and keeping the eggs and nesting area clean is essential in any treatment program. A Vet should be consulted for medication as this disease is often fatal.

Nematodes (Roundworms):

This usually first appears in an infected bird, along with a general lethargy. The presence of eggs or worms in the faeces will confirm infection.

Over-grazing on the same pasture over a period of time can result in the ground being contaminated and so the worms spread quickly through the flock.

Prevention means properly rotating the Geese, so the ground does not become contaminated, along with the usual warnings about sanitation and a clean environment. Geese kept indoors should have their bedding cleaned and disinfected regularly.

Worming tablets can be obtained to expel the worms from the host – be sure to follow the instructions as to the dose etc.

Tapeworms:
Basically the same symptoms as the roundworms; along with the same advice regarding prevention and treatment.

Lameness:

Heavy birds especially can easily become lame. This can be caused by standing on a sharp object, or can be the symptoms of an infection, bumble foot or worms. Treatment involves a close inspection to see that there is no injury to the feet or legs and treating with an antiseptic if necessary.

Worms also cause lameness in waterfowl so worming is a first step and a visit to the vet for an antibacterial injection may be needed.

Coccidiosis:

The symptoms include the bird showing signs of weakness, and a general loss of weight accompanied by blood in the droppings as Coccidia attack the gut linings. This disease is more common in hot wet conditions and can last for weeks rather than days.

Infection is caused by contaminated surroundings, grazing on contaminated grass and by contact with infected birds. Treatment can be obtained from your Vet and usually involves an anticoccidial in the drinking water.

***

Preparing For The Table

If you are NOT keeping Geese for their meat or feathers, then this part may not be relevant for you. However the fact is that there may come a time when you may have to put down an animal for yourself, in order to prevent further suffering.

This must be done swiftly and humanely; and so as distasteful as it may seem to some it is an essential part of animal husbandry, and 'essential knowledge' to anyone seeking to operate their own Homestead or otherwise become self-sufficient in meat production.

Depending on where about on this planet you reside, there may be restrictions as to the keeping and slaughtering of farm animals; I would advise you therefore to inquire to your local authority as to any bylaws regarding this matter.

Preparation:

Before slaughter, Geese and other poultry should be starved for a period of 12-18 hours, with access to water only. This will remove any food from the crop and intestines, thereby removing the risk of contamination when cleaning the carcase.

With regard to Geese and other poultry, there is a simple way to best achieve this with minimal distress to both parties, and this is simply to break the neck by placing the birds head under a broom shaft on the floor, stand either side of the shaft and pull firmly upwards.

Thereafter place the bird upside down in a traffic cone to stop the flapping and cut the throat to bleed the bird. Some people find that the whole episode of the broom-shaft on the floor is a beyond them, and so opt for a straight into the cone, and a quick cut with a sharp knife.

Another option is to stun the bird with an electrical stunner before bleeding; or a firm hit with a blunt object to the back of the head to stun the bird, before cutting the throat.

Admittedly this can be a traumatic experience to many folks, especially if the Goose is an 'Old friend.' I myself once bottled out and sold it at the local market rather than 'do the damage.' It was a Goose called Tom; remember never to name your livestock!

Plucking:

All poultry are best plucked 'fresh' whilst they are still warm if possible. Wet plucking is my preferred method as it is so much easier than plucking the bird dry, where it is possible to rip the flesh without trying too hard!

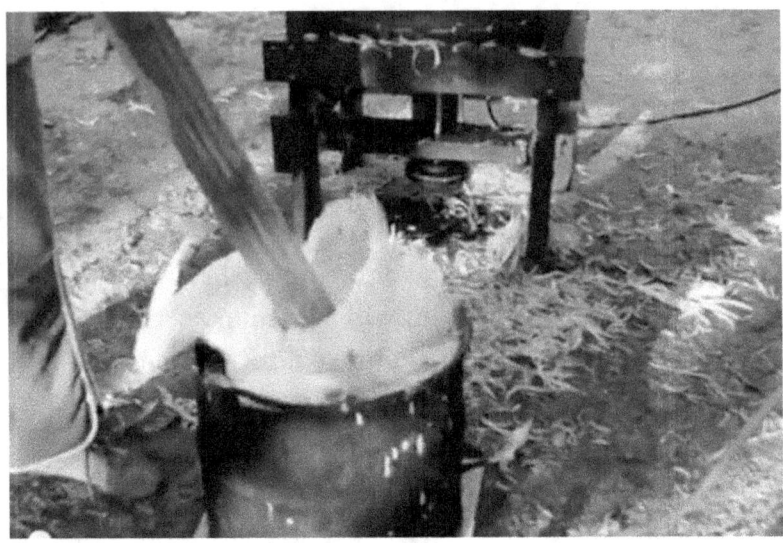

The dry plucking method is simply to pull the feathers from the bird while it is still warm. Starting with the heavy wing feathers and tail feathers, which you will sharply pull straight out.

The body feathers are removed by holding the bird firmly and pulling the feathers 'against the grain' being careful not to tear the bird in the process.
This generally results in a cleaner more attractive carcase; the downside is that it is also easier to tear the skin and is a harder job overall than wet plucking.

The wet plucking method involves heating up a barrel of water to around 60C and dunking the bird into it by the feet for a few minutes. This makes the feathers much easier to remove, with less chance of tearing the flesh. It can however lead to some flesh discoloration, especially if the bird is dunked for too long.

Sometimes it is impossible to remove the pin hairs on the bird, and so a light going-over with a small blowtorch can be used to remove them.

If the feathers are being kept for duvet or pillow stuffing, then this is the time to separate the down and small body feathers from the large wing and tail feathers. The down can be used for the duvet, and the small body feathers for stuffing pillows and the like.

Both should be washed in a gentle detergent; thereafter scattered on a surface covered in a soft porous material in a suitable room to dry out – or sealed into pillow cases and placed in a tumble dryer.

Evisceration:

Simply insert the knife into the vent at the rear, and slit the flesh to the breastbone. Insert your hand high up into the body cavity and pull back to remove the internal organs. Remove the head and cut off the legs at the hock joints.

Wash the bird thoroughly inside and out. If the giblets are to be kept, then wash thoroughly and place into a suitable plastic bag. Place inside the carcase or keep separate.

Freshly killed birds should be dressed as soon as possible, thereafter stored in a fridge for use within 5-7 days.

***

Cooking Goose

Goose is naturally much juicier than Turkey, so at least there is not the same problem with drying out that you have with that particular bird. Also you have the added bonus of Goose fat, which is much prized by top chefs today.

To cook a juicy bird that will serve up to 8 people, you will need a ten pound Goose (4.5kg). Make sure you have a roasting tin that will fit the bird – and that will go into the oven!

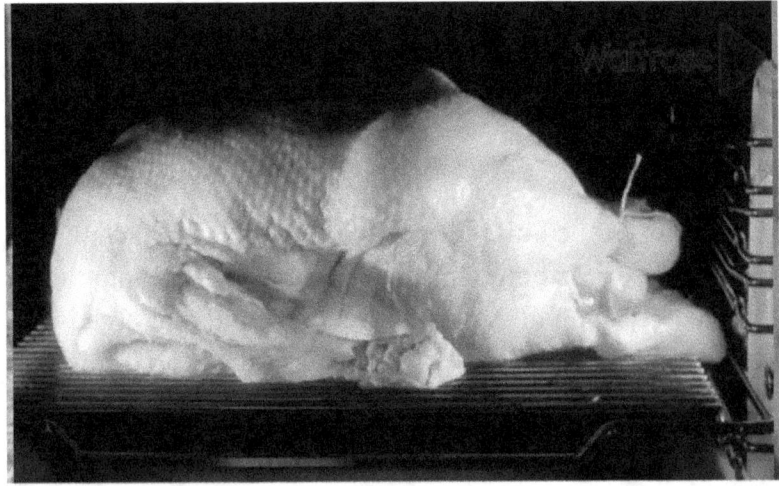

Place the bird in a rack within the roasting tin and set oven to 185 degrees. Cook the Goose for 3 to 3.5 hours or simply follow the instructions for a store-bought bird. Half way through cooking, baste the bird with the fat collected in the cooking tray, and again 20 minutes or so before the set time.

After cooking, rest the bird for 20 minutes or so before carving.

Goose Fat:
Collect the fat from the roasting tray, and strain through muslin or other fine strainer into a Pyrex jug. Allow it to cool then pour into jam jars or equivalent, then store in the fridge.
This is excellent for roasting vegetables like parsnips and other root vegetables, and is certainly the top choice for crispy, tasty roast potatoes!

***

Tasty Duck & Game Recipes

First of all, a big thanks to author F. A Paris for allowing the use of these recipes from her Slow Cooker recipe book 'Slow Cooking Heaven'.

Duck Breast in Orange Sauce

(Serves 4)

Ingredients:

- 4 lean duck breasts
- 3 oranges (sliced)
- 1 small onion (sliced)
- 1 garlic clove (fine chopped)
- 2-3 leaves mint
- 1 tablespoon course marmalade
- 3/4 pint (0.35 ltr) orange juice
- 1 tablespoon honey
- Salt & pepper to taste

Preparation:

Remove any skin from the duck breasts, slice in half and rub over with salt to season.
Layer the duck, onion and oranges in the slow cooker.
Add the orange juice and the rest of the ingredients into a suitable container and mix thoroughly. Pour this mix over the duck in the slow cooker.
Cook on low for 6-8 hours.

When cooked, remove duck and discard the fruit and vegetables, retaining the sauce.

Thicken the sauce to a good consistency with some cornflour or Arrowroot, simmer in a saucepan for 5 minutes or so.

Place duck breasts in a serving dish and pour over the orange sauce.

A delightfully tasty dish served with duck placed on a bed of boiled wild rice. Garnish with slices of Orange.

*****

Rabbit & Red Wine Stew

(Serves 6)

Ingredients:

- 1 Rabbit Jointed & cut into pieces
- 1 large onion (chopped
- 1 clove garlic (crushed)
- ½ pint (0.23 ltr) red wine
- ¼ pint chicken stock
- 1 carrot (sliced)
- 2 oz seeded olives
- 4 potatoes cut into chunks
- 2 table spoons plain flower
- 1 tablespoon cooking oil
- 1/2 oz butter
- 1 tablespoon tomato relish
- Salt & ground black pepper to taste

Preparation:

Coat the rabbit pieces in pre-seasoned flour and add to a hot saucepan with the oil and butter. Turn rabbit pieces until browned all over and add to the slow cooker.

Into the saucepan add the onion, garlic, tomato relish stock and red wine. Bring to the boil and simmer for 4-5 minutes. Pour the ingredients into the slow cooker with the rabbit. Add the other ingredients.

Cook on low for 6-8 hours. Taste, and season with salt, and ground black pepper to suit.

Delightful served with a side of boiled potatoes in butter and oatmeal.

*****

Pheasant with Cherries

(Serves 4)

Ingredients:

- 4 Pheasant breasts
- 7 oz (198g) shallots halved
- 1 jar pitted morello cherries
- 1 large onion (sliced)
- 2 garlic cloves (crushed)
- 2 whole cloves
- 3 bay leaves
- 1 tablespoon honey
- ½ table spoon mixed spice
- 1 table spoon brown cane sugar
- 1/2-pint (0.23 ltr) chicken stock
- 2 tablespoons vegetable oil
- ½ oz butter
- Salt & pepper to taste

Preparation:

Coat the pheasant breasts with well-seasoned flour, and fry with the oil and butter in a saucepan for 4-5 minutes. Remove and add to the slow cooker.

Add the shallots, garlic and sliced onion to the saucepan and fry for 2-3 minutes, then add the rest of the ingredients. Bring to the boil and simmer for 4-5 minutes before adding the mix to the slow cooker.
Cook on 'low' for 2 ½ - 3 hours.
Taste, then season/thicken to suit.

Can be served with boiled rice, or potatoes and vegetables, to make an ideal evening meal.

*****

Pheasant with Pancetta & Sweet Chestnuts

(Serves 4)

Ingredients:

- 4 Pheasant breasts
- 7 oz (198g) whole peeled chestnuts
- 7 oz shallots
- 3 ½ oz (99g) smoked sliced pancetta
- 1 teaspoon French grainy mustard
- 2 sliced apples
- ¼ pint (0.11 ltr) sweet cider
- ¼ pint chicken stock
- 1 garlic clove (fine chopped)
- 1 tablespoon tomato relish
- 2 table spoons plain flour
- 1 oz butter
- Salt & pepper to taste

Preparation:

Dry the pheasant then season well with salt & pepper; wrap the pheasant in the pancetta, holding in place with string or cocktail sticks pierced through the meat. Add to a hot saucepan along with the oil and butter. Fry for 3-4 minutes. Remove and add to the slow cooker.

Into the hot saucepan add the shallots, chestnuts, garlic, stock and the other ingredients. Bring to the boil and simmer for 3-4 minutes, then add to the slow cooker along with the pheasant.
Cook on 'low' for 2 ½ - 3 hours, then season to taste.

Very satisfying dish if served with roast & mashed potatoes & vegetables. Or with a simple base of basmati rice.

*****

Venison & Cranberry Stew

(Serves 4)

Ingredients:

- 1 lb (450g) venison loin (cubed)
- 1 onion (chopped)
- 1 clove garlic (crushed)
- 5 oz (141g) cranberries
- 2 oz (56g) mushrooms (sliced)
- 1 carrot (chopped)
- 1 tablespoon tomato relish
- 2 sprigs rosemary

- 1 tsp mixed dried herbs
- ½ pint (0.23 ltr) brown ale (Guinness?)
- ¼ pint (0.11ltr) beef stock
- 2 tsp grainy mustard
- 2 tsp brown sugar
- 2 table spoons plain flour
- 1 tablespoon vegetable oil
- 1 oz butter
- Salt & black pepper to season

Preparation:

Coat the diced venison in well-seasoned flour and add to a saucepan with the oil and butter. Fry and turn the meat to brown all sides, then remove and add to the slow cooker.

Add the onion and garlic to the pan and fry for 2-3 minutes, then add the mushrooms, rosemary, mustard, herbs, tomato relish, brown sugar, stock and brown ale to the saucepan. Bring to the boil and simmer for 4-5 mins.

Add the mix to the slow cooker along with the sliced carrots. Add seasoning.
Cook on 'low' for 7-8 hours, taste and season as required.

Fantastic stew for a cold winters evening, served with a creamy mash and green beans.

*****

Conclusion:

As mentioned earlier, there are a number of good reasons for keeping Geese, including for meat, eggs and feathers as well as just for pets. Admittedly there is no economic argument for keeping them for eggs, as even the best layers will only produce around 40 or so eggs per year.

That aside, the eggs that they do produce, I have always looked on as a kind of bonus as they are difficult to purchase in most stores – and expensive even if you can find them for sale.

The Christmas Goose is quite rightly making a come-back, and gaining some ground on the Christmas Turkey. Both birds in my opinion have their place on the dinner table – and not just for Christmas.

***

Authors Note:

I hope you have found these books on keeping Ducks and Geese, to be as informative as you expected, and trust that you will put the information in this introductory work to good use!

Homesteading, or simply the desire to live a more sustainable or self-sufficient lifestyle, is becoming of more and more importance as people in general are becoming disenfranchised with the commercialization of every aspect of their lives – and with good reason.

With so many chemical fertilizers promoting rapid fruit and vegetable growth, toxic pest control methods, additives and preservatives added to processed foods to improve the shelf life; it is maybe time we all took a little more control over our food intake at the least!

In this Homesteading series, and the shorter introductions in my Homesteaders K.I.S.S series, I hope to introduce many aspects of self-sustainability – from growing vegetables to rearing a selection of animals synonymous with the Homestead.

Finally – A HUGE THANKS for purchasing this book!

Thanks again,

Norman

***

www.ingramcontent.com/pod-product-compliance
Lightning Source LLC
Chambersburg PA
CBHW071106240526
45469CB00006BD/2345